Newborn 101

The Essential Guide for New Parents to Raise a Healthy Baby

Table of Contents

Introduction

Congratulations on downloading this book and thank you for doing so.

The following chapters will discuss some of the topics that new mothers want to know about when bringing home their newborns. This is an exciting time in your life, and you are ready to bring home that little baby and start your new life with them. But despite all of this excitement and your happiness, it can still be a time of concerns. Mothers may be worried about how to breastfeed, how to get through labor, how they can prepare for the baby, how to take care of their baby when they first bring the newborn home and so much more.

It is perfectly natural to ask all of these questions and being prepared ahead of time can make it easier to take care of your baby later on. This guidebook will provide you with some of the answers you need to properly take care of your newborn. We will talk about how to prepare your home, the stages of labor, how to make breastfeeding easier, ways to soothe your baby when they are fussy, and even when it is time to call the doctor over one of your concerns.

Every new parent has questions and concerns about taking care of their babies. With the help of this guidebook, you will have all of the information that you need to gain confidence so you can spend less time worrying and more time bonding with your new baby.

There are plenty of books on this subject on the market, thanks again for choosing this one! Every effort was made to ensure it is full of as much useful information as possible, please enjoy!

Chapter 1: How to Prepare Your Home

You can even start preparing yourself and your home before the baby arrives. This is the perfect time to get a head start on some cleaning, baby proofing and organizing before you have those sleepless nights and a baby to take care of. Taking care of some of the essentials ahead of time can help you to remain calm once the baby comes home because you won't have so many worries running through your head. Here are a few of the things that you can do to help prepare yourself and your home for your new baby.

Feed yourself

Once you bring home that baby, there isn't going to be a lot of time for preparing meals, and you don't necessarily want to spend a lot of money going out all of the time. Preparing ahead of time so you and your family will have food for the first few weeks is important to ensure that you stay healthy and have the energy that you need.

There are a few ways that you can do it. You can purchase some freezer meals to have on hand for when you are too tired to cook. You can prepare some of your own freezer meals as well, which is a lot healthier and will even save you money. Some families will purchase a few gift cards so they can grab something easy when they feel hungry.

Feed the baby

If you are choosing to breastfeed your baby, make sure that you purchase a high-quality pump. You can either purchase one (many insurance companies will help with this now), or you can rent a hospital grade one. Consider a nursing pillow as well because this will make both you and the baby more comfortable. Even with breastfeeding, consider having some bottles on hand for when you send the baby to daycare, or you are interested in letting others feed the baby at times.

Try to get some sleep

This one is easier said than done in most cases, but getting enough rest, especially when this is your first baby and you don't have others to chase around, is so important. Many mothers during the last trimester have trouble getting enough sleep because they are uncomfortable, they may have aches and pains, or the baby is moving around a lot. But even just taking it easy will help you out and prepare you for when the baby comes.

It will not be long before your baby arrives, and the long days and nights will start to catch up to you. It is best to get as much sleep as possible during this time, but taking things slowly, such as not working out as hard, taking some time off work, and just relaxing at night, can make things so much easier to handle and will rest your body up before baby gets here.

Setting up the baby's room

Take some time to set up the room for your baby. Whether you are keeping the baby in their own room or in your room for a bit, there are a few things that you can do. Start out by making the room a little bit darker. The baby will take naps during the day, but this can be hard when the room is bright and sunny. You can get some light canceling curtains to help and keep some lights inside of the room down to a minimum. Having some white noise or soft music in the room can be nice as well.

In addition to making sure that the room is comfy and dark for a sleeping time, you also can organize some other things. Hang up and put away the clothes that you have gotten for the baby. Set up the crib and make sure that the sheets are on properly. Store the other supplies that you have gotten such as diapers, bath supplies, wipes, toys, book and more. Get everything organized ahead of time to help put you at ease.

Smooth out the edges

Edges need to be taken care of before the baby is born. If there are any edges that you are worried about, it is time to smooth them out. This can be on the sides of walls, on door frames, on furniture and so on. Take a few moments to go through the house and see where some of the edges are. Imagine how you would feel if you ran into one of these, and then determine if you would like to smooth them out. These edges are going to be dangerous once your little one starts moving around, which will be sooner than you can imagine, so take care of those edges before the baby arrives.

Secure moveable furniture

Take a look around your home and see if any pieces of furniture can easily be moved. Do they shake a bit and would they be an issue if the baby started grabbing onto them when they begin walking? If there is any furniture that can move around or topple, it is time to secure it properly. Make sure that shelving is hooked up to the wall, that you put some stoppers on couches, and secure down anything else. The shakiness of a shelf or something else may not seem like a bit deal right now, but you never know what the baby will get ahold of, and it is always best to be safe.

Finish up some projects

If there are some projects that you want to get done around your home, now is the time to work on them. You are not going to have this time once you bring the baby home. So spend some time finishing them up. Whether that includes painting the baby room, cleaning out the cabinets, or you have some other project you and your partner have been discussing, now is the perfect time to work on it. You would be surprised at how quickly time can go after the baby comes and it could be a few years before you get back to them.

Pack your hospital bags

If you are planning on delivering the baby in the hospital, make sure to pack up a hospital bag ahead of time. You do not want to try to do this while you are in labor and with the bag all ready to go, you can just grab the bag when you are ready to go to the hospital. There are a few things that you can add to the bag. Include some outfits for the baby and some diapers and wipes. Pack some clothes and toiletries for yourself as well since you will most likely spend a few days in the hospital as well. Bring some magazines, a computer, or anything else that you would need to make yourself as comfortable as possible in the hospital.

Get the car seat

Remember that the hospital is not going to let you take your new baby home until you have a car seat and they are able to see that it is properly installed inside of your car. This can seem like a hassle, but it is meant to keep the baby safe along the way. They will be able to help you learn how to buckle the baby in the car seat and will help you learn how to take the base in and out in case you need to do this before you leave the hospital. Make sure that your car seat is not only safe, that it hasn't gone past its expiration date (you should be able to find this on the bottom of the seat), and that it is installed properly.

Chapter 2: Getting Through Labor

Probably the one thing that makes new mothers the most nervous about having a baby is getting through labor. They can plan for pretty much anything else that happens, but they worry about the pain, and the whole process, is something that is hard to prepare for. This chapter will discuss some of the most important aspects of going through labor so you can understand what is happening to your body and how you can prepare as much as possible ahead of time.

Setting up a birth plan

Before you go into labor, it is a good idea to discuss a birthing plan with your doctor or your midwife. This birth plan is just going to be a clear, usually just one-page, statement that will list out your preferences during the birthing process. You should provide a copy of this plan to anyone who will be involved with the birth but do discuss it with your health care provider to make sure they are on board as well.

Work on this plan ahead of time to make sure that you aren't as stressed out about it as you would when waiting until the last minute. There are a lot of things that you can place on this birth plan, but try to keep it simple. You can list out who you would like to be present during the birth, do you want medication, do you want skin to skin contact right after birth, if you will allow fetal monitoring, and so on.

Of course, you do need to make sure that you keep some form of flexibility. Things do happen, and sometimes the doctor will have to make some changes during the delivery of this birthing plan. Having this birth plan can help to answer questions when you are in labor and not in the best position to explain yourself, but having flexibility will ensure that you get the best experience for you and your baby.

The stages of labor

No matter how much you talk to other mothers or read up on labor, it is truly something that you have to experience to understand what it is about. It is completely different for everyone, and it is really hard to explain what labor is about. But understanding some of the different stages that come with labor will make it easier for most mothers. While we can't get rid of the pain that comes with labor and we can't tell you how long the labor pains are going to last, sometimes knowing exactly what to expect will make all the difference. So let's take a look at the three stages of labor and determine what is going to happen during each one.

First stage of active labor

To keep things simple, the first stage is going to start when you feel your first contraction and will go until the cervix has had time to dilate to 10 centimeters. It is the longest stage of the birthing process, and a lot of things do happen with it, but it is pretty much going to be the stage until you start pushing that baby out. This first stage is going to start at home, and when it is done, you are within a few minutes of seeing your new bundle of joy. The length of time this first stage of labor is going to vary; some mothers will see it last just a few hours and others will see it last for a day or more.

When this stage starts, you should expect some regular contractions that will last around 30 to 45 seconds. They can feel like really strong menstrual cramps or like a backache depending on what type of labor you are dealing with. In the beginning, the contractions are going to be mild, and they could end up being 30 minutes or so apart. As the labor goes on, the contractions will become a lot closer together and so much stronger.

Many mothers wonder about their water breaking. Some mothers will have the water break early on, and others could be pushing the baby out when the water breaks. It can technically break anytime during your first stage. You should take a note about when it breaks, but this act is not something to worry about because your delivery may be awhile off still.

We are going to assume that your bags are already packed to go to the hospital, so all that you need to do during this stage is to just try to relax. Taking a bath, getting a back rub, listening to music, or even trying to eat can help keep your mind off the contractions a bit. This process is allowing your cervix to open slowly, and you could have a good 12 hours or more of them before you call up the midwife or go to the hospital.

When you start to feel that the contractions are becoming regular and closer together, it is time to keep track of them. When they start to last for about 40 to 60 seconds, and they are four minutes or less apart, going from the start of one contraction to the start of another one, you should make sure that your midwife is on hand or that you head to the doctor. At this point, depending on the mother, you could be somewhere between 4 and 7 cm and the contractions will just get stronger.

If you go to the hospital, they will likely admit you over to a birthing room, and you will be hooked up to monitors to measure the heartbeat of the baby and the strength of the contractions. If you had agreed to get pain medications, this is the time when you will start to get them.

From here, you will probably stay in a pattern for a bit longer. It will probably be similar to one minute of contractions that are pretty strong and then a few minute rest, and it will be on repeat. You can still work with some of your distractions rather than sitting around and feel worried about each contraction. Thinking about things that will keep you calm, doing some deep breathing, and more will really help with this.

This is the part that gets really difficult, and it is important that the people you keep in the room with you are going to be there to keep you calm. You can use pain management drugs if you would like, but some mothers choose to forgo this as well.

As the cervix finishes up to opening to 10 cm, the contractions are going to start being on top of each other. You may hardly get any breaks in between so finding distractions will be hard. The good news is that you are in the final part of it all and soon everything will be over. This intense stage of labor is the final leg of the race, and it rarely lasts more than an hour.

Stage 2: the big push

For this stage, your cervix has reached 10 cm and is completely dilated. This means that the mother needs to start pushing. You are going to have some contractions, but these are helpful guides to show you when it is time to push. The pain you feel will slowly start to move down your body as the baby is pushed out. The good news is that while pushing can be difficult, it does come naturally. Your body already knows that the baby needs to come out, so it is ready to go.

The amount of time that you take to push will greatly depend on how much medication you get. Those who took epidurals can take up to two hours to push the baby out, but it can be as short as twenty minutes as well. You will need to take quick rests between the pushes so you can be ready for the next stage. You will finally be at the end as soon as the baby crowns.

Once the baby is finally out, your health care provider is going to check the baby's health and will cut the cord. If the baby is healthy, the nurses around you will clean them off, wrap them off, and let you hold your new baby. It is even possible to begin nursing right after the birth too. Some medical centers will even let you hold onto your baby because clamping and cutting the umbilical cord so that you will not have to wait for too long.

Stage 3: the winding down stage

At this point, your baby is in your arms, and the hard work is done, but there is a little bit more to finish up. You will still need to deliver the placenta. This is usually done within ten minutes, but can sometimes take a bit longer. You will feel a few contractions as the placenta works to separate from the uterine wall, but they are pretty mild compared to what you just went through. The doctor can help finish this by massaging your stomach. You may notice that once the placenta is delivered, you will shake or shiver a bit. Don't worry about this because it is just a natural response to delivery for many new mothers.

If you were not progressing properly with dilating the cervix or your doctor and you discussed it beforehand, you may go with a C-section. This is usually going to require you to spend a few more days in the hospital than before. Vaginal births can usually go home between one to three days, and C-sections will go home within three to five days depending on the complications that may arise. If everything goes smoothly, you get to go home sooner.

Chapter 3: Those First Few Days at Home

Congratulations! You have given birth to your baby, and now it is time to bring them home. While the pain of labor is now done, there is a whole new set of worries that you need to concentrate on. It is completely natural to be a little concerned about how you and baby will do when you first get home. At the hospital, you had professionals there to help you any time that you needed a break, had a question, or when a concern came up. But at home, it is time to get into your own routine and learn how you and the new baby will start a life together. This chapter is going to give you some tips to help you out during those first few days at home with your newborn.

Breastfeeding

Many mothers choose to start breastfeeding their babies, and this can start right away in the hospital. Breastfeeding is all natural, provides the best nutrients for your baby, and can be convenient. But this doesn't mean that there are not a few challenges that occur in the process. Some of the tips that you can follow when you are ready to start breastfeeding includes:

- Seek help when needed: mothers who looked for help with breastfeeding were those who saw the most success out of the endeavor.
- Use resources at the hospital: you have a ton of professionals around you in the hospital, why not ask questions while you have them there
- Prepare: keep things on hand for you to do, such as some water and a book to read. Breastfeeding can take some time to be prepared.
- Warm compresses: your breasts can feel sore and sometimes they will become engorged. A heating pad can help with this and can help with the milk flow.

Sleeping

For the first few weeks, if your baby isn't eating, they are probably asleep. Some newborns will sleep for 16 hours at a time, but remember this is in bursts and not all at once. This can make a new mother really tired and figure out how to deal with the sleep deprivation can be hard. Some of the things that you can do to help with this include:

- Don't obsess over being tired: your main goal right now is to take care of that baby. You will not get the sleep you want so don't even think about it right now.

- Take shifts: you and your partner should take turns with the baby, so you both get a chance to get some sleep.

- Sleep when the baby sleeps: this is a good piece of advice, especially if you don't have other kids. Both of you can go to bed early or take a nap together.

- Do what works for you: in the first few weeks, don't worry so much about forming habits; those can come later. Let your baby fall asleep on your chest, in the car seat, while rocking or whatever else works.

Soothing

At some point, you will need to be able to soothe your new baby and make them calm down. In the beginning, you may be unsure about what will help them to stop crying or being fussy. Some of the things that you can try out include:

- Mimic the womb: swinging, holding the baby on their sides, shushing, and swaddling can all mimic how the baby felt in the womb and can make them comfortable.

- Play tunes: something calming, like classical music, can help to keep a baby nice and calm.

- Soak them: a warm bath can sometimes soothe your baby down as well.

- Try something else: each baby will be different, so try something out of the box and see what works.

Staying sane

You may be super excited to be a new mommy, but all of the cares that your infant requires can be really draining. Finding some ways to take care of yourself, and learning how to lower your expectations a bit so you can steal short breaks can be so important. Some of the things that you can do to stay sane during this stage include:

- Forget the housework: concentrate on just getting to know your new baby. If someone has a complaint, point them to the cleaning supply closet.
- Accept help: if someone is offering, they truly do want to help. Whether it is bringing you a meal, holding the baby so you can take a shower, or something else, let them do it.
- Reconnect: join a mom's group, go to the store, or do something else that will get you out of the house and see other people.
- Pick the bigger jobs: the diaper change really only takes a few minutes. See if those offering to help will take on a bigger job like sweeping the floors, bringing a meal, or even running to the store for you.

Taking the baby out

If the weather permits it (or you are brave enough to bundle them up and go out anyway), it is a good idea to go out and about with your new baby. Whether it is on a walk, going to visit friends, or making a trip to the store, getting out of the house can be so nice. Some of the ways that you can make this easier includes:

- Enlist some help: take someone you trust with you the first few times you go out. They can help provide you with support and keep you on task.
- Stick to places that like babies: some places are more baby friendly than others. A book store, a library at story hour or some other choice can work nicely.
- Keep the diaper bag ready: there is nothing that is worse than getting your baby all ready to go when you still have to grab your own stuff.
- Keep extra clothes around for you and baby: you just never know when you may need them.
- Embrace the craziness: it is going to be crazy the first few times you go out, so just start to expect this, and things will be easier.

Those first few weeks with a baby are going to be chaotic, and you may be uncertain about what to do at times. But if you take things easy and don't expect things to be perfect, things will work out so much better than you can imagine.

Taking the baby to their first appointment

If you feel that this is going to be too much for you to handle in the beginning, there is some good news. The first doctor's appointment is going to come up shortly after you bring the baby home, and this is a great place to air your concerns and to ask questions that you may have. For the most part, your pediatrician will want to see the baby within a few days after they head home from the hospital.

At this first visit, the pediatrician is going to perform a physical examination to make sure that the baby is healthy and happy. This will include a height and weight check. You can also ask questions and discuss concerns. Make sure that you are putting your baby in clothing that is pretty easy to take off and bring along a blanket so that it is easier for them to get weighed in the process.

Pediatricians will not only answer the questions that you may have during this appointment, but they will also ask a lot of questions, such as about your home life and the schedule you are starting with the baby. They may want to know how other kids in the family are doing with the baby or they may ask questions to figure out if the mother is tired, run down, depressed, or overly stressed.

It is very important for you to have good communication with your health care provider. This ensures that your baby is getting the best care possible for their situation. Most pediatricians want this open communication, and they are very open to you contacting them with any concerns or questions that you may have, especially during the first year.

One way to prepare for this first visit is to make sure that you have some questions ready. Since you are likely to be very tired from taking care of a baby, put the list in the fridge and add to it any time that a new question comes up. Then you can just grab this list and head out the door whenever you are ready for that first appointment.

Chapter 4: Tips to Make Breastfeeding Easier

When you bring your baby home, there are two options for feeding your baby. Some people choose to go with formula. They may not want to worry about how breastfeeding will go, or they like the convenience of using the formula so that their partner is able to help with feedings at night. They may even be concerned about going back to work, and they just want to stick with the formula.

Others will choose to breastfeed. While breastfeeding is a great option to go with, it is all natural, has all the nutrients that the baby needs to stay healthy, and it is less expensive than formula, some challenges come with using his option. It is important that new mothers are set up understanding what breastfeeding is all about and the challenges that they may face along the way.

Most people know about all of the benefits that come with breastfeeding. They know that this milk is going to contain all of the nutrients that the baby needs in the right balance. They know that breast milk is easier for the baby to digest compared to commercial formula and that the antibodies that are found in breast milk will boost the immune system of the baby.

Breastfeeding can even be beneficial to the mother, helping her to lose weight, bond with her baby, and so much more.

Even knowing all of this, some challenges can come with breastfeeding. Your supply may take some time to come in, or you may have trouble making enough to satisfy the baby. Your baby may have trouble latching on or learning how to go with this method. Your breasts may become inflamed or sore from the activity, and it can be really hard to breastfeed when you have to go back to work, and pumping is not that easy or comfortable either.

With all of these concerns, it is no wonder that some new mothers are worried about breastfeeding their newborns. They want to provide their newborns with all of the benefits that come with breast milk, but they are also worried about adding more stress and worries that are already there. If you are considering breastfeeding, here are some of the tips that you can follow to help make this whole process easier.

Ask for help

Reading online and in books about breastfeeding is a good start, but trying to do it all on your own can be the big challenge. The first time that you breastfeed the baby, which will usually be shortly after delivery if it is possible, make sure to ask for help. There are usually nurses and a lactation consultant available in the hospital who are able to offer tips, such as showing you how to position the baby and to help you learn how to do the latch properly. This is the best place for you to learn because there will be a lot of people around who can help you.

When you get started, you will need to make sure that you are comfortable. You can even support yourself with some pillows if you need. Cradle your baby close to the breast, but do not lean forward and try to bring the breast to the baby or you will be really uncomfortable. Support the head of your baby with one hand and then support your breast with the other one. With your nipple, tickle their lower lip to encourage the baby to open up their mouth wide. The baby will then take in part of the darker area near the nipple, and the nipple should be far back in the baby's mouth. Listen for a swallowing and sucking pattern that is rhythmic from your baby.

If you want to switch the baby around to the other breast, you can release the suction. Don't just pull off though because this can really hurt. Take your finger and gently insert it into the corner of your baby's mouth. This will release the suction so you can move them.

Let the baby pick the pace

For the first couple of weeks, your baby is going to breastfeed every few hours, day and night. Watch for some of these early signs of hunger to know when it is time to breastfeed. As you start to become familiar with your baby, you will catch on to these signs easier, but look for lip movements, sucking motions, restlessness, and stirring.

Let the baby nurse from the first breast completely, until it starts to feel soft. This will take around fifteen minutes, but remember that there is not really a set time. Some babies will take longer, and some will take shorter. When they seem like they are done with that breast, try to burp them. You can then offer them the second breast. If the baby is hungry after the first breast, they will latch on to the second breast and continue to eat. If they are not hungry, you just need to start the next session on that other breast.

Sometimes the baby will only want to breastfeed on one of your breasts. This is fine, but consider pumping with the other breast to relieve some of the pressure and to make sure that your milk supply stays up.

Let the baby sleep in your room

For the first few months at least, let the baby sleep in your room. This helps to lower their risk of SIDS, and it can make feedings at night so much easier. Do not let them sleep in your own bed though because they could become trapped and even suffocate on the bed. This can be from the mattress or sheets on the bed or from the parent rolling over on them. Put them in their own bassinette or crib so that they are safe, but still nearby.

Keep the pacifier away

Some babies will be the happiest when they have something to suck on, even when it is a pacifier. But for some babies, if you give them a pacifier too soon it can interfere with breastfeeding since sucking on this pacifier is going to be different than sucking during breastfeeding.

According to the American Academy of Pediatrics, you should wait until you have established a good breastfeeding routine before you introduce in a pacifier. Pacifiers are not all bad because when a baby sucks on one during bedtime or naptime, it can reduce their risk of SIDS. You just need to make sure to introduce it at the right time, so it doesn't interfere with your breastfeeding efforts.

Take care of the nipples

In some cases, even if you do everything correctly, your nipples can become sore and uncomfortable. There are a few things that you can do to make this better. After the feedings are done, it is fine to let milk dry on them because this helps to keep the nipples soothed. You can also change out the bra pads in between feedings if you have some leaking because this can get uncomfortable. When you bathe, make sure that you keep the soaps, cleansers, and shampoo down to a minimum because this will irritate the nipples more during breastfeeding.

If your nipples end up becoming cracked or dry, make sure that you use a form of lanolin after each of the feedings. These will help to moisturize your nipples and make them feel better, and it is completely safe for the baby.

Make good choices

You also have to take care of yourself when it comes to breastfeeding. Everything that you do will affect the breast milk that you are providing to your baby, so you do need to take some precautions. Some of the things that you can do to ensure that you make good lifestyle choices include:

- Eat a healthy diet with lots of nutrients
- Drink lots of water, milk, and juice
- Get as much rest as possible
- Don't smoke
- Be cautious with your medications

Breastfeeding is a great way to provide food and nutrition for your baby and for you both to bond together, but succeeding with breastfeeding can be a challenge. When you learn how to give it some time and follow the other tips in this chapter, you will be able to provide the very best to your baby without quite as much hassle.

Chapter 5: How to Soothe Your Baby Back to Sleep

As a new parent, you are going to be tired. You want to provide the best for your baby, but you were up going through all the labor and delivery process, and that little bundle of joy is not on a regular schedule of letting you sleep through the night. Dealing with this lack of sleep can be hard for any parent, whether they are with their first child or they are going through this again.

Getting frustrated when your baby won't fall asleep is not the best answer, yet it is so easy for new (and sleep-deprived parents) to feel like things are hopeless. In many cases, this is going to make things worse. The baby will start to feel that you are getting anxious or upset, and that will make things worse. That is why the first step that you need to do anytime that you are trying to soothe your baby back to sleep is to just remain calm. If you can't do this right then (and there will be times when this happens), trade off with your partner for a few minutes to regain yourself.

Once you are sure that you are calm and ready to handle the situation, there are a few other things that you can try out to help soothe your baby down, so they go back to sleep. Some of the tricks that you can try out include;

- Make sure the baby is dry and fed: no baby wants to go to sleep if they are hungry or wet and they are going to cry. This may seem obvious, but when you are sleep-deprived, it is easy to forget these simple things. Make sure to check their diaper and see if they want something to eat and see if this will help.
- Hold the baby: many times, your baby just wants you to hold onto them. You love your baby, and they love you too. They sometimes just want to be comforted, to have their parents hold onto them for a bit. You can't spoil your baby in the first few months, so there is nothing wrong with holding them to help them feel comforted at night.
- Rock the baby: the back and forth movement that you do while rocking can be really comforting to the baby, especially when you are holding the baby. Even a few minutes of this can help your baby calm down.
- Take a walk around the house: sometimes the baby wants a different movement. Something may be bothering them with the rocking, or they want to take in some different scenery. Do a quick walk around the house and see if this is the result that the baby needs.
- Try some music: for some babies, some gentle music is able to ease up the tears a little bit. It can calm them down, distract them a bit, and many babies like to have some soft noise instead of all the silence around them. You can pick out a CD that you like to do this when you aren't in the room or signing works great too.

- Pat or rub their back: as you are holding onto your baby, try to rub their back, either in a circular motion or going up and down. Some babies like to have their back patted. This rhythmic patting can mimic the heartbeat, which is a sound that the baby is very used to so it will be calming to them.

These soothing strategies are pretty simple to work with, and often doing one or two of them will be enough to get the baby to calm down and go back to sleep. You do have to learn what is going to work the best for your baby. Some may like walking around more while others are better with some music or singing. As you become more comfortable with your baby, you will quickly learn what works the best for you.

If you have tried out a few of these options and they are not working, and you are starting to become more frustrated, it is time to take a break. Never get so overworked that you may cause harm to the baby. It is fine to set the baby down in their crib, even if they are still crying, and then walk out of the room for a few minutes to calm down. Yes, they are still crying, but they will be fine while you regain yourself enough to go back into them.

Chapter 6: The Importance of Self-Care Postpartum

Now that we have taken some time to talk about the ways that you can take care of your newborn once they come home, it is time to talk about how you can take care of yourself a little bit. Many new parents get so involved in taking care of the baby that they forget they need some care as well. While you may be missing out on some of that sleep you are used to at this time, it doesn't mean that you can't work to take care of your body and your mind in other ways. And in reality, if you don't provide some all important self-care to yourself, you are going to start falling behind in the care you provide your newborn. Let's take a look at some of the things that you can do to ensure that you make self-care a priority, even when you are taking care of the baby.

Making it a priority

The best thing that you can do when you are expecting your new little one is to make sure that you and your partner sit down and go over the expectations that you have for each other. This is the time when you will need to tell your partner that you have to schedule in some self-care time. You may both decide to hire in a housekeeper to come in and clean once a week to help out, you can ask people you know to bring in some meals during those few weeks, or to hire a doula. You can agree that each night the mother gets to go take a bath or go for a walk by herself to clear her head or do something else special.

It doesn't matter what type of plan you come up with, the important part is that it becomes a priority. Waiting until the baby is born is not the best idea because emotions are going to be high and both partners will be low on the sleep they need to think rationally.

Lower your levels of stress

During that first couple of weeks, you should try to make sure that you are spending some time doing something for yourself each day. It doesn't have to be that complicated or take that long. Something like taking a few moments to drink some coffee, doing some journaling, reading a bit in a new book, or taking a shower. Find something that doesn't take a long time (that you can sneak in during nap time if needed) and will still make you feel good when it is all done.

In addition to doing something small each day, you should find a way to schedule a "mom day" at some point in the first few months. This is something that allows you to get out of the house on your own for a few hours. It can be refreshing to get out without the baby for a little bit, and this special day gives you something to look forward to. Some of the things you can consider doing includes leaving the baby with someone so you can get a nap, getting your hair or nails done, going to pick out a new outfit, read for a few hours in a bookstore, and so much more.

Get some sleep

As a new mother, you will probably hear all the time that whenever the baby sleeps, you should sleep. This is great advice, but in practice, it doesn't always work out that way. It is hard to fall asleep when the baby is napping. You are probably going to think about all of the things that you could be doing, such as making supper, cleaning the house, and more.

Despite the long to-do list that is running through your head, it is still important to stop and get some sleep. Your body is running on way less sleep than it is used to at this point in the game and this can really mess with your mood and your health. So any time that you are able to sleep, go ahead and do it. When someone comes over, let them hold the baby while you go and take a nap. Let your husband take care of the baby so you can get some sleep. Ignore the dirty dishes and other chores for a bit; no one really cares about these when they come over and if they do, invite them to take over the mess.

Things will get back into the routine that you are used to, and you will get those chores done. But as a new mother, your job right now is to be well rested so you can take care of that baby. So, make sure that you are getting as much sleep as possible.

Eat right

Yes, this one is going to seem impossible right now. You are already so busy taking care of a newborn and so tired from it all that the only thing you are thinking about is finding food that is fast and doesn't make you spend all day in the kitchen. But it is important to your recovery that you eat healthy foods that are good to the body and to the brain.

Healthy fats need to be a priority in your diet because they are a hormone and brain food. They will help you to feel so much better compared to just grabbing something to eat out all of the time. Remember that one of the biggest risks to postpartum depression is a diet that is poor, so you will need to pick out a diet that will help feed the body in the right way.

This can be hard which is why you should prepare ahead of time. Making some freezer meals to keep on hand for those days when you just can't get to supper can be nice. You can just pull out one of the bags and have dinner ready, with the added bonus of knowing the food is always healthy and yummy for you.

Get some movement

This does not mean that you need to get right back to your strenuous workout routine that you were doing before you got pregnant. This is actually bad for you. You need to give your body some time to recover after having a baby so take things slow. But sitting around on the couch all day long is not really the answer either.

Getting a little bit of activity each day will help you to feel better in no time. Just put the baby in their stroller and walk around the block a few times a week. Consider finding an easy yoga routine so that you can begin stretching a little bit at a time. The movement will help you to recover more and can increase your mood after having a baby, but you do need to remember to take it slowly during your recovery time.

Reduce risk of postpartum depression

It is so important to prioritize self-care and rest during those first few weeks after having a baby. If you start out making new habits out of this, it is going to be easier for you to stick with this and get the results that you want, rather than trying to build up a new habit later on.

When you take the time now to take care of yourself, you will find that you are less stressed, will have much lower blood pressure, and you can even have more energy to put towards your new mothering duties. All of these can help you reduce your risk of postpartum mood disorders. If you are not able to give yourself some of the self-care that you need, it is going to be hard to give your baby the care that they need.

Self-care is so important for a new mother who is recovering. This is a part of bringing home a new baby that many new mothers will forget about or put on the back burner, but it is still so important to work with. Take some time for yourself, try to get in some movement (even if it is just a quick walk around the block), let others help you out, and try to eat healthy meals, and you will be amazed at how much easier it is to take care of your newborn.

Chapter 7: How to Take Care of a Preterm Baby

When a baby is born before they reach the 37th week, they are going to be considered premature and often will be called preemies. This is a new territory, something that you may not have been counting on when you did all of your planning before bringing this new baby home. Most mothers who bring home a preemie baby will b nervous and scared because these babies will have more risks of complications due to being born early.

The complications that could arise are going to increase the earlier that your baby is born. Any of these complications are going to be addressed by professional nurses and doctors in the NICU, or the neonatal intensive care unit. As a new parent, it is important to know what to expect when it comes to taking care of a preterm baby and what your role will be during this time.

Premature babies are not completely ready to deal with life outside of the womb. Their bodies are still going to have some parts that are undeveloped including the immune system, digestive system, skin, and lungs. The part that still needs to develop will often depend on how early the baby was born.

This can sound pretty scary, and you may be worried about how the baby is going to be able to survive outside the womb. The good news is that thanks to medical technology, it is possible for preemies, even those born extremely early, to live until they are strong enough and are developed enough to do all of this on their own.

There are several ways that a preemie will come. Sometimes the body will decide that it is ready to give birth before it is time and the mother is going to feel contractions and the other signs of labor. Often, when the mother gets to the hospital, they will be able to stop the labor and will put her on bed rest in the hopes of keeping the baby in the womb for a bit longer. Sometimes they may not be able to stop the labor, and the baby will be born early.

On the other hand, sometimes the doctor will decide that it is in the best interest of the mother and of the baby to have the baby be born early. There are some conditions, such as elevated blood pressure in the mother, that could make it dangerous for both if the baby stayed in the womb, so it is better for the baby to be born. Your doctor will be able to discuss this with you ahead of time.

Whether your baby is born a few weeks early or a few months early, a premature baby can be a scary experience, and most new parents are not ready to deal with this. The time that the baby is born early will also determine how long they will have to remain under care in the NICU.

The NICU is going to be the new home and protective environment for the baby for a little while. It is a good idea to become familiar with this place so that you know what is going on, who is doing what, and how you should play a role in this area. The NICU is going to have everything that your baby needs to continue developing and to be ready to go home with you including access to physicians in every specialty, respiratory equipment, monitoring systems, and caring staff.

If you have never spent time in the NICU, all of the equipment that is found inside can sometimes seem a bit overwhelming and even scary, especially if this was not a planned thing and you are just out of surgery after giving birth. Learning how all of these machines work will make it easier to relax and will prevent you from getting scared and nervous.

The staff in the NICU will be your best resources to helping you understand these machines and equipment. Each hospital is a bit different, but there is basically going to be every piece of equipment that is needed to help your baby grow big and strong. The staff will spend a lot of time with your baby and you, helping you to understand what is going on and helping to make sure that the baby is developing properly so familiarize yourself with them and don't be afraid to ask them questions if you have these.

Kangaroo Care

One type of care that you may be interested in is known as Kangaroo Care. This is a technique where a preemie baby is going to be placed on the mother's bare chest, in an upright position, so that there is tummy to tummy contact between the baby and the mother. The head of the baby will be turned so its ear can be right at the heart of their mothers.

Numerous studies show how this kind of care can greatly help and benefit the baby. Some of the ways that Kangaroo Care can help the preemie baby includes:

- Increased intimacy and bonding: this is so important no matter the baby because it helps them to feel safe.
- Increased weight gain: this kind of care is going to make it easier for your baby to fall into a nice deep sleep, which means that they can take that energy and direct it towards other functions of the body. When the baby increases their weight gain at a faster pace, it means they will stay in the hospital for a shorter amount of time.
- Breastfeeding: this kind of care means that the baby will have easier access to the breast, which will help them to grow. This kind of skin contact will also make it easier for milk production to come in.

- Body temperature: studies have shown that baby's and mothers will have thermal synchrony. So, if the baby is feeling cold, the mother's body temperature can help to warm them up.

All of this is important to help the baby grow and prosper while in the NICU. Baby needs to have a warmer temperature, the ability to gain weight faster, and even more intimacy so that they feel safe and secure in this new setting. When all of this comes together with the help of Kangaroo Care, it is easier than ever for your baby to get healthier and move out of the NICU faster.

How can you help?

As a new parent of a preemie baby, you may feel like you are at a loss for what you should do. You want to be there to support your baby and to help them grow, but you may also feel like anything that you do is going to hurt them or won't work the way that you want. While your professional doctor and nursing staff may take over a lot of the medical stuff that your baby needs, it is encouraged for the mother and father to interact as much as possible with the baby.

There are quite a few ways that you are able to interact with your baby and help them to become stronger along the way. Some of the options that you have available include:

- Touch the baby as often as you can. Stroking motions, holding their hands, holding them with Kangaroo Care, or any other option will work really well.
- Talk to the baby. Your baby is already able to recognize your voice, and it is going to be very comforting for them to hear you. You are not just limited to talking to the baby, it is fine to sing or read to the baby.
- Change your baby's diaper, read to them, or do some other regular day things.
- Be there for their first bath. You may have to use sponges or washcloths depending on how your baby is doing.
- Help out with some of the procedures for your baby. This can include simple things such as taking their temperature.

Dealing with the NICU can be a bit scary, and many new parents are not sure how to handle it. The good news is that you can be very involved with the care because this is going to help your baby be ready to go home earlier. Depending on how early the baby was born, it can take them some time to get to come home with you. You can work with your doctor to determine the right milestones that need to be hit so your baby can go home.

Chapter 8: Bringing Home Multiples

When you find out that you are having twins or more, things are going to be a little bit different. Yes, you will still have some of the same challenges that other mothers have, but now some of those issues are going to be multiplied. For example, just because those two babies look alike doesn't mean that they are going to have the same eating or sleeping schedule.

But the day has finally arrived. You and the multiples are ready to come home. It may have seemed like forever while you were pregnant (that anxiety and worry that comes from carrying multiples can make time drag on), but now it is time to bring them home. Your multiples may already be a few weeks old or more depending on if they needed to stay in the NICU due to their early birth, but the same kind of preparation can be done either way. Take in a deep breath, realize that you may need some more help than other parents and that no matter what, you will be able to adjust to this new life in time.

First things to consider

When you are bringing home your babies, you need to make sure that you have infant approved car seats. Each state is going to have some different safety standards so make sure that you check on these before purchasing both car seats. You will need one for each baby, and often it is recommended that you purchase them new to make sure that they aren't damaged or compromised in any way. You will need to make sure that these are installed in the car properly. Finding a specialist to help you with this, perhaps before you need to bring the baby home, so you are not under pressure so that you know they are in properly.

Getting the home ready

You will be able to follow some of the advice that we gave earlier about preparing your home for one baby, but you may have to take some extra considerations and do a little extra work to prepare for two babies. There will be a lot of equipment that you need, but not all of it is needed right away. For example, your babies will not need a high chair right away since they are not able to sit up on their own so you can hold off on this until later.

When picking out some of the supplies that you will use, consider whether you will actually need two of each thing. Many parents of multiples think that because they are having twins or triplets that they need to have that many of each thing. This can get really expensive and is not really necessary. For example, you are probably still fine with just one swing because one baby may rock to sleep in it while the other one is eating or eating on the floor. There are very few times when both babies will want to be in the same contraption at the same time.

Another thing that you will need to have is a place for your babies. You will need to consider whether you want to place them in their own cribs and get them used to that right away or if you want something that will allow them to sleep in your room and is a bit more temporary for now. Doing a twin bassinet can work well to hold the babies in your own room, but at some point, you will want to get them their own cribs as well.

When it comes to picking out a place for the babies to eat, you won't need to work with a high chair right now because they are too little and these chairs are going to take up a lot of space. In the beginning, you may be just fine getting a comfortable chair for yourself for feeding them. Make sure the chair is big enough, so you are able to feed both babies at once if you need.

Keep a lot of the babies' cleaning supplies on hand. This would be things like wipes, diapers, and plenty of changes of clothes. One baby can make a big mess so imagine what two or more are able to do. It is sometimes hard to figure out how many diapers you are going to need ahead of time in each size, so stocking up is a bit of a challenge. If your babies are born early, it is possible that they could stay in the small sizes for a few months. But sometimes these babies can grow fast just like any other baby, and they may need a bigger size a lot sooner than you thought. This means that you will need to keep lots of diapers on hand, but try not to overbuy on them either.

While we are on the subject of diapers, you should consider having a diaper disposal, especially when we are dealing with multiples. You can get a diaper container that contains odor, so your home will still smell good. This is totally optional though because many families will save money on this, and will just throw the diapers into some plastic bags.

Get some help

When you are bringing home more than one baby at a time, there is going to be a big need for help. It is tough to do this all on your own because you have twice as much work. Your babies will not sleep at the same time or even stay on the same schedule so it can be tough to ever find time for a break for you to get to sleep at night. So before you bring these babies home, it is a good idea to think about the type of help that you want to have.

In most cases, you will be able to find people who are willing to help, and they may already be offering. But it is also important to never be afraid to ask for help when you need it. People want to be there for you, and you are not doing yourself or your babies any favors by trying to do it all on your own. Most of the time people will be thrilled to help you out, so keep a list of those who offer to help and then take them up on that offer whenever you need.

Sometimes, you may need to be direct in what you need for help. Rather than waiting for someone to offer, tell them exactly what you need. If you need an errand done, care for older siblings, pet car, meals prepared, or someone to watch the kids so you can take a nap, make sure to tell others. People are often willing to help, especially when they know your hands are full with multiples, but they may not know what would help you out the most.

Things to consider:

As a parent of multiples, there are a few things that you should consider when you bring these new babies home from the hospital. Some of these considerations include:

- You may not be able to bring both babies home at the same time. Sometimes one baby will have more complications than the other after birth, while the other one is ready to go home. This can seem hard, but there are some ways that will make the adjustment easier. If you only need to care for one baby to start with, it will give you a bit of time to catch your breath along the way.

- You do not need to do everything right this second. Some parents get obsessed about childproofing their homes before the babies even get home. But your baby will not be moving all around the home for at least a few months. You do need to do it before they move around, but it doesn't have to be your top priority right now.

- If the babies are born early, or they have other special needs, be aware that there could be some extra medical issues that come up in addition to the normal requirements that come with taking care of an infant. You should work with the caregivers for your babies to make sure that you learn the proper way to take care of these babies.

- Many times, multiple is going to be born smaller than other babies. This means that some of the outfits you got as gifts or purchased may not fit in the beginning. You may have to rely on preemie clothes, even if they are only born a few weeks early, to help keep them warm.

- Work up to having a schedule. Your babies are not going to be on a good schedule right from birth, and you are working with two, rather than one. You will eventually find a schedule that works for both you and the babies, and it is fine to stick with this one. You can work to get them on the same schedule, but don't worry about whether that schedule makes a lot of sense to other parents.

- Learn how to get to know the babies. Some parents are worried that they will not be able to tell their babies apart, but this is often easier than you can imagine, especially if you take the time to bond and connect with your babies. You will be able to pick up on their personalities and even their cries pretty quickly.

Bringing home multiples can be really challenging for new parents. You may be overwhelmed by what you need to do and how you are going to be able to handle these two different personalities at the same time. But when you learn how to take your time, relax, and provide them with the care and attention that they need, and you will be just fine.

Chapter 9: Common Concerns with Your Newborn

As a new parent, it is common to have a lot of questions and concerns about how to take care of this baby. Here we are going to take a look at some of the common concerns that parents will have about their newborn and some of the steps that you can take to make sure you get through these hard times.

How can I encourage my baby to sleep?

Getting your baby on a sleep schedule can be difficult, and there really isn't a magical way that you can get the baby to fall asleep. But there are a few things that you can try. The first thing to consider is a bedtime ritual for the baby. It isn't reasonable to just expect your baby to fall asleep on their own. Most of the time they will need a bit of a routine to help them out. Playing with them a bit, giving them a bath, getting them warm and comfy, and then rocking them to sleep can really help the baby to relax and fall asleep.

There are a few other things that you can try out as well. You can try to lull them to sleep with a bottle or by breastfeeding, but don't let them fall asleep with this in their mouth to help prevent ear infections and tooth decay. Try out a few different sleeping arrangements to see what is most comfortable for the baby; they may like to sleep in the room with you. And always look to see if there is something that is causing them to have trouble with sleeping, such as being too cold or too hot.

How can I prevent SIDS?

Many new parents are worried that they will lose their babies because of SIDS. While it is pretty rare to occur, it is a high worry for most parents. There are a few things that you can do to help prevent SIDS in your baby though, including:

- Provide a healthy environment in the womb: low birth weight and premature birth are two big risks for developing SIDS. Getting good care during pregnancy and eating right will help with this.
- Keep smoking away from the baby: this is considered one of the biggest risk factors for developing SIDS. Make sure that you do not smoke around the baby and keep other smokers away.
- Keep the baby on their back: when the baby is awake, tummy time can help them develop stronger muscles. But at night, the baby needs to sleep on their back.
- Make sure that the environment that you provide the baby to sleep in to help keep SIDS away.

How can I keep my baby healthy, they seem to get sick often?

Some babies seem to get sick more often than other children, and this can be hard for a new parent. There are a few things that you can do to help keep your baby healthy and to prevent them from catching every cold and flu that comes along:

Breastfeed as much as possible: babies who get breast milk are less likely to get sick. And even when they do get sick, it is not as severe.

Keep their nose clear: if the baby's nose gets clogged, get some nasal drops and use a nasal aspirator to help clean them out. This helps to keep the infections out.

Keep your home and the sleeping environment clean: when their sleeping environment is clean, it is easier for the baby to stay healthy.

Take them to their doctor visits: this is the best way to make sure your baby stays healthy. It will ensure that your baby gets the immunizations that they need to stay healthy.

When should I discipline by child

When you have a baby, it is not really about disciplining your baby, although you are starting to build the bonds of trust and showing your baby the right way to behave. For example, when you childproof your home, you are setting limits on where the baby is allowed to play. When you say no, you are helping the baby learn when they are headed for trouble. You should not discipline your child really at this time, just concentrate on getting some of the right boundaries.

How will I be able to balance a job and parenting

Many parents choose to work outside of the home after their baby is born, but this can cause a lot of tension and worry for a new parent. They want to still be there and form those attachments to their baby, but they still need to leave home to earn an income. The good news is that there are a few things that you can do to make sure you keep those close bonds, even when you have to head back to work:

- Share the work: if both of the spouses in your home have to work, it is important that both parents will take on some household chores so that they can both spend time with the baby as well.
- Happy departure and reunion: before you head off to work, cuddle the baby and make them feel good, and then do the same thing once you come home. If you are breastfeeding, let the caregiver know that they should not feed the baby right before you get home so that you can use this as your bonding time.
- Attachment time: when you are with the baby, it is fine to use attachment time. You can use a baby carrier when you are cleaning or doing errands so that you and the baby get plenty of time together.

How do I get my spouse to help out more?

You thought you were getting into this together, but now it seems like you are the only one who is doing all of the work. This can make it hard for a tired mom to take on all of the work. Sometimes it is simply because your spouse needs to be taught how and when to help out. The first thing that you can do is to choose the tasks that you need a lot of help with and then do them with your partner. Pont out the techniques that work for you, but let them have a chance to try out things on their own.

You should also consider letting dad be home all alone with the baby at times. You will be surprised in most cases about how well dad can do on their own. If you are breastfeeding, make sure to feed the baby before you go or leave some milk behind to help him out. And then when dad is dealing with the crying baby, don't just come to the rescue all of the time. Let them have some time to work it out on their own sometimes.

Is my baby getting enough nutrition?

It is hard to tell sometimes whether your baby is getting the right amount of nutrition to stay healthy. This is why it is helpful to go to the doctor when required because they are able to track the baby's weight and will tell you. Then after a few months, you will be better able to tell if the baby stays healthy or not.

Let's take a look at the breastfed infant. By the time the baby is a week old, a well-fed baby who is breastfeeding will have about six wet diapers a day with a few stools. If you feel that the milk is letting down, and you hear the sucking and swallowing noises, it is likely that your baby is going to be getting plenty of nutrition. It is pretty normal for a baby to lose some weight when they are born, but they will gain it back pretty quickly if they are getting the right nutrition. You can visit with your pediatrician to determine if the baby is getting the right nutrition along the way.

It is sometimes easier to tell if the bottle-fed infant is getting the right amount of nutrition. As a newborn, they only going to take about two ounces at each feeding, but by the first month, they may be up to four ounces. A good rule of thumb is that your baby will take in about two ounces of formula each day for each pound they weigh. So if your baby is 10 pounds, they will probably take in about 20 to 30 ounces each day.

Conclusion

Thanks for making it through to the end of this book, let's hope it was informative and able to provide you with all of the tools you need to achieve your goals whatever they may be.

The next step is to start following some of the tips that are in this guidebook. Some of these are going to be pretty easy to implement, and you can even get started on a few, such as preparing your home, before the baby is even born. As a new parent, you are sure to have a lot of questions and concerns, and this guidebook is going to help you learn how to take care of your baby and yourself, without feeling too overwhelmed.

This guidebook is the guide that all new parents need to read to help them prepare before their baby arrives. We will talk about how to prepare your home, how to get ready for labor, how to get through those first few days of having the baby home including how to help them sleep and how to breastfeed, and even how to take care of yourself. There are also sections about how to take care of a preemie baby and what to do when you bring home multiples.

When you are expecting a new baby, and you want to make sure that you are as prepared as possible, make sure to read through this guidebook to learn everything that you need.

Finally, if you found this book useful in any way, a review on Amazon is always appreciated!

9 781979 615242